# THE WEIGHT LOSS CODE

## (WORKBOOK)

Lose Weight & Keep It Off
On Your Terms And At
Your Pace

ISBN: 978-1-8381760-3-7

Cover design & layout by: Worital Global (hello@worital.com)

THIS WORKBOOK BELONGS TO:

NAME:

PHONE:

EMAIL:

IF FOUND, PLEASE RETURN TO:

ADDRESS:

# A SUCCESSFUL WEIGHT LOSS JOURNEY, AT LAST!

Thank you for getting 'The Weight Loss Code Workbook' and well done for taking the next step in your weight loss journey. Shifting from contemplation to concrete plans and action is one of the first steps to a successful weight loss journey, so you are already on the right path by purchasing this workbook.

I am passionate about helping you to succeed on your weight loss journey, so I have put this workbook together to enable you to implement the weight loss tips and strategies you will discover in my book – The Weight Loss Code: A Practical Guide to Sustainable Weight Loss.

In the pages that follow, you will find everything you need to complete the activities in the book, including templates to help you assess your current weight status, to set your weight loss goal, to plan your meals and exercises, and lots more that will guide you on your way. In short, you will receive everything that will take you from your 'here and now' to your desired 'there and then'.

This workbook is simple to use and navigate, but if you need support at any point, have questions, or better still, if you want to share your success stories, feel free to reach out to me on any of these platforms. I always love to engage with my readers.

Facebook:
*https://www.facebook.com/Booksbyyemifadipe*

Twitter:
*https://twitter.com/YemiFadipe4*

Instagram:
*https://www.instagram.com/booksbyyemifadipe/*

Email:
*weightlosscode@yemifadipe.com*

I wish you the very best and I cannot wait to hear your success stories.

# THE WEIGHT LOSS CODE BUNDLE

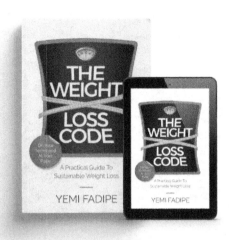

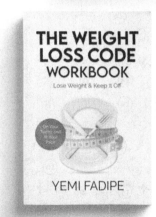

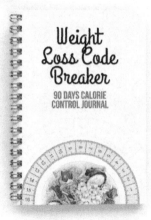

# CONTENTS

# LET'S GET STARTED
## How to get the most out of your workbook

Here is a quick guide to help you to correctly navigate and make the most of your workbook.

**Step 1:**
Order your copy of 'The Weight Loss Code – A Practical Guide to Sustainable Weight Loss'. You will find The Weight Loss Code in electronic and paperback format on ***Amazon, Google Playbook, Bambooks.io*** or ***Okada books.***

**Step 2:**
Take a couple of minutes to flip through the chapters and pages of your book. Each section has a set of activities, which are set out in grey boxes throughout the book.

**Step 3**
Also, take a few more minutes to familiarise with this workbook. You will find that it's specifically tailored around the content and activities in 'The Weight Loss Code' book. . Your workbook is where you will be completing the activities you come across as you read through The Weight Loss Code book.

## Step 4

Begin reading your book. Feel free to skip the dashboard section of this workbook and start from Chapter 1 – you will be signposted back to the dashboard pages at a later stage.

## Step 5

Complete all activities in each chapter before moving onto the next section in your book. To complete each activity, return to the corresponding chapter in your workbook and use the template provided.

## Note:

This workbook should not replace your weight loss app. However, you may find that your app already has some of the tools or trackers that I have included in this workbook e.g., the weight trackers. Some pages may be more relevant to you if you are tracking your weight loss progress manually, so if you decide to stick to your app instead of using the book as well, that's absolutely fine.

A PDF copy of your workbook can also be downloaded for a minimal fee from
*www.weightlosscode.co.uk*

# YOUR
# WEIGHT LOSS
# DASHBOARD

# KNOW YOUR CURRENT WEIGHT STATUS

*As catchy as it might sound to ask you to begin with the end in mind, firstly, you need to know where you are right now.*

- Visit the NHS BMI calculator (https://www.nhs.uk/live-well /healthy-weight/bmicalculator/).
- Record your current height and weight and use your results plus the additional information requested to determine your current BMI.
- Be honest when doing this as we will be using this information shortly to set your target.

Date: .........................................

I am ................ (ft, in/cm) tall and currently weigh ................ (kg/st/lb)

My BMI is ...........................................

**My Current Weight Status:**

Underweight ☐  Healthy Weight ☐  Overweight ☐  Obese ☐

# WEIGHT LOSS
# COMMITMENT

I commit to:

*(insert your goal statement. This is your end goal and not the milestones in between now and then.)*

I commit to an end goal of below 200 lbs.
I commit to exercising by walking each day building up stamina.

*E.g. I commit to losing X kg/lb every week for the next X months to achieve a weight of X kg/lb and a BMI of 22 by exercising for 1hr daily and controlling my calorie intake.*

Sign ........................................

Date: ........................................

# MILESTONES – CELEBRATE SUCCESS

*You can break down your end goal into smaller, more achievable goals (milestones) and tackle each stage one step at a time, celebrating your successes while keeping the END GOAL in mind.*

- Set your weight, BMI, or body measurement milestones below, and when you reach each milestone, return here to record your achievement date and celebrate your success.

| WEIGHT | BMI | BODY MEASUREMENT | ACHIEVED |
|---|---|---|---|
| | | | |
| | | | |
| | | | |
| | | | |
| | | | |
| | | | |
| | | | |

CHAPTER 1

# MIND-SET FOR SUCCESSFUL WEIGHT LOSS

# THE 3 D'S OF WEIGHT LOSS

*There are three essential ingredients for weight loss and maintaining a healthy body weight: Decision, Determination and Discipline. Without them, any weight loss regime or diet plan will become an unsustainable waste of time.*

My strongest D is ⋯⋯⋯⋯⋯⋯⋯⋯⋯⋯⋯⋯⋯⋯⋯⋯⋯⋯⋯

I have applied my strongest D in my everyday life to achieve the following:

1. ⋯⋯⋯⋯⋯⋯⋯⋯⋯⋯⋯⋯⋯⋯⋯⋯⋯⋯⋯⋯⋯⋯⋯⋯⋯
2. ⋯⋯⋯⋯⋯⋯⋯⋯⋯⋯⋯⋯⋯⋯⋯⋯⋯⋯⋯⋯⋯⋯⋯⋯⋯
3. ⋯⋯⋯⋯⋯⋯⋯⋯⋯⋯⋯⋯⋯⋯⋯⋯⋯⋯⋯⋯⋯⋯⋯⋯⋯

How will I apply this strength to my weight loss journey?

⋯⋯⋯⋯⋯⋯⋯⋯⋯⋯⋯⋯⋯⋯⋯⋯⋯⋯⋯⋯⋯⋯⋯⋯⋯⋯⋯⋯

⋯⋯⋯⋯⋯⋯⋯⋯⋯⋯⋯⋯⋯⋯⋯⋯⋯⋯⋯⋯⋯⋯⋯⋯⋯⋯⋯⋯

⋯⋯⋯⋯⋯⋯⋯⋯⋯⋯⋯⋯⋯⋯⋯⋯⋯⋯⋯⋯⋯⋯⋯⋯⋯⋯⋯⋯

⋯⋯⋯⋯⋯⋯⋯⋯⋯⋯⋯⋯⋯⋯⋯⋯⋯⋯⋯⋯⋯⋯⋯⋯⋯⋯⋯⋯

⋯⋯⋯⋯⋯⋯⋯⋯⋯⋯⋯⋯⋯⋯⋯⋯⋯⋯⋯⋯⋯⋯⋯⋯⋯⋯⋯⋯

## What will I do differently to boost my other Ds?

.................................................................................................

.................................................................................................

.................................................................................................

.................................................................................................

.................................................................................................

.................................................................................................

.................................................................................................

.................................................................................................

.................................................................................................

.................................................................................................

.................................................................................................

# KNOW YOUR 'WHY'

*Know your WHY and tap into it. Whatever your reason is, make sure it is something that can keep you motivated. Having a goal in mind helps you to picture where you are heading.*

What is/are your whys? (Begin with the most important reason for losing weight. E.g., I want to be healthier as I age, or I want to fit into a smaller size of clothing.)

#1. I want my weight to stop being the cause of health issues!!

#2. Picture Kim G. 74 yr. old matheson TV, cute clothes – classy sportswear. I want to be older & have a style.

# I need stamina to do whatever work God wants me to do.

CHAPTER 2

# YOU ARE
# ALLOWED
# TO EAT

# KNOW YOUR NUTRIENTS

*There is no bad food as such. The nutrients we need to remain healthy come from varied food groups.*

+ Whether our quick detour through basic nutrition was an update for you or new information, try the little exercise below now that you understand more about the role of nutrients.

+ Relook at the foods listed as sources of each nutrient and create a list of foods you have excluded from your diet in the past or considered "bad" food.

| FOOD | NUTRIENT CLASS |
|------|----------------|
|      |                |
|      |                |
|      |                |
|      |                |
|      |                |
|      |                |
|      |                |
|      |                |
|      |                |
|      |                |

Which nutrient(s) have you deprived your body of and what could be the consequence to your body and your health? Find out more here:

***https://www.healthline.com/health/malnutrition***

.............................................................................................................................

.............................................................................................................................

.............................................................................................................................

.............................................................................................................................

.............................................................................................................................

.............................................................................................................................

.............................................................................................................................

# CHAPTER 3

# CALORIE CONTROL 101

# WHAT'S ON MY PLATE?

> *Sustainable weight management is not achieved by food or nutrient deprivation. Portion control is essential, and it needs to be combined with a healthy balanced diet.*

+ Set a day (or days) aside to confirm your current breakfast, lunch and dinner portion sizes.

+ Before each meal:
    + Make a list of the food/ingredients in your meal. Retain packaging or take photos of the front and back of each label. You will need them for another activity later.
    + Weigh the empty plate and write down the result.
    + Dish up your meal as you normally do.
    + Weigh the dish of food and write down the result.
    + Subtract the weight of the empty plate from the weight of the plate of food. The difference is the weight of each meal.
    + Write down the weight of your breakfast, lunch and dinner for that day on the meals table shown.

+ Using the calories information on your labels, insert the food/ingredients from the list you created into their relevant categories on the calorie density table provided. Feel free to repeat for other food/ingredients you use regularly.

## MEAL TABLE

| Date | Meals | | Weight /Portion Size |
|------|-------|--|----------------------|
| | Breakfast | | |
| | Lunch | | |
| | Dinner | | |
| | Breakfast | | |
| | Lunch | | |
| | Dinner | | |
| | Breakfast | | |
| | Lunch | | |
| | Dinner | | |

# CALORIE DENSITY TABLE

| High Calorie Density >4 kcal/g (>113kcal/oz.) | Medium Calorie Density 1.5-4 kcal/g (43-113kcal/oz.) | Low Calorie Density 0.6 – 1.5 kcal/g (17-43kcal/oz.) | Empty Calories <0.6 kcal/g (<17kcal/oz.) |
|---|---|---|---|
|  |  |  |  |
|  |  |  |  |
|  |  |  |  |
|  |  |  |  |
|  |  |  |  |
|  |  |  |  |
|  |  |  |  |
|  |  |  |  |
|  |  |  |  |
|  |  |  |  |
|  |  |  |  |
|  |  |  |  |
|  |  |  |  |
|  |  |  |  |
|  |  |  |  |
|  |  |  |  |
|  |  |  |  |
|  |  |  |  |
|  |  |  |  |
|  |  |  |  |

CHAPTER 4

# SMART
# SWAPS

# SMART SWAP
# CHALLENGE

*Indeed, you can eat whatever you like, but depending on how soon you want to reach your target weight, you may need to swap some high calorie foods for their lower calorie equivalents. Switching to lower calorie food stretches your daily calorie budget, allowing you to get more food for less calories.*

+ Create your own Smart Swaps for the high calorie density foods in the list you created in the previous activity.

+ Use the calorie checkers in the tools and resources page to find lower calorie alternatives.

+ Decide what to swap, and mark as Swap, Cut, or Swap and Cut.

**Swap:** an outright change to a lower calorie alternative.
**Cut:** is where I keep the same food but reduce my level of consumption.
**Swap & Cut:** is where I swap to a more nutritious alternative but still reduce my level of consumption because the calorie content on a like-for-like weight is still comparable.

| Food/ Ingredient | Kcal Per 100g /per serving | My Smart Swap | Kcal Per 100g /per serving | Calorie Savings |
|---|---|---|---|---|
| e.g. Butter | 744 | Light sunflower spread | 289 | 45.5kcal per serving **(Swap)** |
| | | | | |
| | | | | |
| | | | | |
| | | | | |
| | | | | |
| | | | | |
| | | | | |
| | | | | |
| | | | | |
| | | | | |
| | | | | |
| | | | | |
| | | | | |

| Food/ Ingredient | Kcal Per 100g /per serving | My Smart Swap | Kcal Per 100g /per serving | Calorie Savings |
|---|---|---|---|---|
| | | | | |
| | | | | |
| | | | | |
| | | | | |
| | | | | |
| | | | | |
| | | | | |
| | | | | |
| | | | | |
| | | | | |
| | | | | |
| | | | | |
| | | | | |
| | | | | |
| | | | | |

# CHAPTER 5

# EXERCISE: WHERE DOES IT COME IN?

# EXERCISE PLANNING

*Exercise is where the third of our 3D ingredients comes in handy – DISCIPLINE. Adults between the ages of 19 and 64 should be physically active daily and engage in at least 150 minutes of moderate intensity physical activity every week. Be sure to seek medical advice first if you have any underlying health issues.*

+ Look up different forms of exercises. Select your top five and think about what you need for each (kit, equipment, clothing, fees/subscriptions, time etc.). In short, count the cost and list what you need to get started.

+ Using the exercise research template provided, order that list from the lowest cost to the highest. You may find that your favourite is the highest cost (money and time) to you. That's not a problem.

+ Choose the two you can start the soonest and easily obtain everything you need for them (exercise kit, accessories, and clothing).

+ Use the weekly exercise plan template to draw a simple schedule of when you can carry out this exercise: the time of day and for how long. For example, daily from 6.30am to 6.40am, or 5pm - 6pm etc.

## EXERCISE RESEARCH

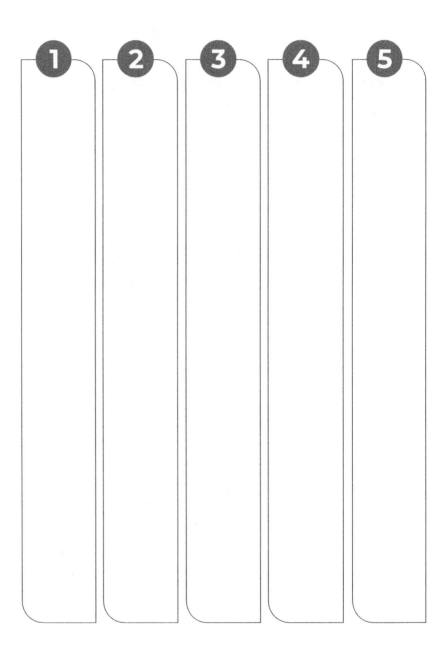

# WEEKLY EXERCISE PLAN

| DAY | WORKOUT | DURATION |
|-----|---------|----------|
|     |         |          |
|     |         |          |
|     |         |          |
|     |         |          |
|     |         |          |
|     |         |          |
|     |         |          |
|     |         |          |
|     |         |          |
|     |         |          |
|     |         |          |
|     |         |          |
|     |         |          |
|     |         |          |
|     |         |          |

CHAPTER 6

# SET YOURSELF
# UP TO SUCCEED

# READY - STEADY - GO

*Successful weight loss is about DOING. We are now going to start the calorie control lifestyle. You would create a list of the tools you need and how to get them. Get your phone or laptop because you will be downloading, bookmarking, and creating a shopping list.*

+ Now you know the main things you will need, but there will be other minor things to pick up as and when needed. Can you go ahead and complete your shopping list before we move forward?

+ Search the play store/app store or the internet and choose your preferred app using the information above. Ensure you select a calorie control app.

+ Create your account and download the app. Alternatively, set up your paper-based system using the templates provided in the next activity.

# SHOPPING LIST

## GROCERIES

- ☐
- ☐
- ☐
- ☐
- ☐
- ☐
- ☐
- ☐
- ☐
- ☐
- ☐
- ☐
- ☐
- ☐
- ☐
- ☐
- ☐
- ☐
- ☐
- ☐
- ☐
- ☐

## TOOLS & UTENSILS

- ☐
- ☐
- ☐
- ☐
- ☐
- ☐
- ☐
- ☐
- ☐
- ☐
- ☐
- ☐

## EXERCISE TOOL KIT

- ☐
- ☐
- ☐
- ☐
- ☐
- ☐
- ☐
- ☐

# SHOPPING LIST

## GROCERIES

- ............................................................ ☐
- ............................................................ ☐
- ............................................................ ☐
- ............................................................ ☐
- ............................................................ ☐
- ............................................................ ☐
- ............................................................ ☐
- ............................................................ ☐
- ............................................................ ☐
- ............................................................ ☐
- ............................................................ ☐
- ............................................................ ☐
- ............................................................ ☐
- ............................................................ ☐
- ............................................................ ☐
- ............................................................ ☐
- ............................................................ ☐
- ............................................................ ☐
- ............................................................ ☐
- ............................................................ ☐
- ............................................................ ☐
- ............................................................ ☐

## TOOLS & UTENSILS

- ............................................................ ☐
- ............................................................ ☐
- ............................................................ ☐
- ............................................................ ☐
- ............................................................ ☐
- ............................................................ ☐
- ............................................................ ☐
- ............................................................ ☐
- ............................................................ ☐
- ............................................................ ☐
- ............................................................ ☐
- ............................................................ ☐

## EXERCISE TOOL KIT

- ............................................................ ☐
- ............................................................ ☐
- ............................................................ ☐
- ............................................................ ☐
- ............................................................ ☐
- ............................................................ ☐
- ............................................................ ☐
- ............................................................ ☐
- ............................................................ ☐

## READY OR NOT?

+ Smart Swap shopping list completed ☐

+ Tools & utensils shopping list completed ☐

+ Exercise toolkit shopping list completed ☐

+ All orders placed and shopping done ☐

+ All orders delivered ☐

+ All equipment (e.g. exercise equipment, scales) set up ☐

+ Decided on preferred calorie system/app ☐

+ Purchased my journal/Downloaded my app ☐

Now this stage has been completed, we are ready to dive in. How are you feeling about this?

Pessimistic ☐  Nervous ☐  Not Sure ☐  Positive ☐  Excited ☐

If you are unsure/nervous/pessimistic, examine why and be sure that you have carefully thought through the D's you need to get through this journey.

# SET YOUR GOAL

+ Visit the NHS BMI calculator again.

+ This time, under activity level, select 'active' or 'moderately active', depending on your exercise plan.

+ Play around with different body weights until you find the weight range that puts you in a healthy BMI (green).

Current Weight: ................ Health Weight Range: ................

Current BMI: ................ Healthy BMI Range: ................

My Current Weight Status:

Underweight ☐ Healthy Weight ☐ Overweight ☐ Obese☐

**Specific:** ................

*(Specify what you want to achieve)*

*E.g. I would like to achieve a healthy BMI, size 16 to 12, etc.*

**Measurable:** ................

*(define a measurable indicator of your progress and what success will look like?)*

*E.g. I would like to lose X kg/lb to achieve a BMI of 22.*

## Achievable: ....................................................................................................

*(what you will do to ensure that you make progress towards your goal. This can include setting key milestones)*

*E.g. I would like to lose X kg/lb and achieve a BMI of 22. I can achieve this by losing X kg/lb weekly.*

## Realistic & Reasonable: ..........................................................................

*(how you can successfully execute your plan given your current circumstances and resources at your disposal)*

*E.g. I would like to lose X kg/lb and achieve a BMI of 22. I can achieve this by controlling my calorie intake and exercising for 1 hour daily to help me lose X kg/lb weekly.*

## Time bound: ....................................................................................................

*(set a deadline for when you intend to achieve your goal)*

*E.g. I would lose X kg/lb every week for the next X months to achieve a weight of X kg/lb and a BMI of 22 by exercising for 1hr daily and controlling my calorie intake.*

## Write out your SMART goal below:

........................................................................................................................

........................................................................................................................

........................................................................................................................

........................................................................................................................

........................................................................................................................

........................................................................................................................

*Go back to the Commitment page and write down your weight loss commitment and the milestones you have set for yourself based on this smart goal.*

# SET YOUR DAILY CALORIE BUDGET

## USING AN APP

Once you have decided on your end weight goal, set your target in your app. In my app, this was under Goals>Details> Configure>New Program. You will be presented with a range of plans based on weekly weight loss (0.25kg, 0.5kg, 0.75kg, 1kg or maintain current weight) and the corresponding realistic end date. Choose what works for you, and you are ready to go!

You should now see your daily calorie allowance on the app. As you log your meals, daily exercise, and update your weight as it changes, the app will adjust your daily calorie allowance accordingly.

## PAPER BASED APPROACH

If you are using a paper-based system, complete this activity using the template provided on the next page.

+ Simply decide how much weight you need to lose per week to reach your target by the deadline you have set in the previous activity. For example, if your end goal is to lose 4kg and your deadline is in 4 weeks, then you want to lose 1kg per week.

+ To set your daily calorie budget/allowance, you will need to create an account with one of the apps we used above. Alternatively, you can use the online calorie calculator available at ***https://www.calculator.net/calorie-calculator.html***

+ Record your calorie budget on the template provided.

+ Unlike using an app, you will not be able to benefit from the automatic calorie adjustment, so you need to get into the habit of checking and updating your calorie budget regularly at set intervals. For example, at every 2.5kg (5.5lb/0.5st) weight change.

## CALORIE BUDGET TRACKER

*You will only need to use this paper-based tracker if you are using a paper-based system, otherwise your app will automatically track this for you. Record your current daily calorie budget below. Get into the habit of checking and updating your calorie budget and your weight.*

| Date | Body Weight | Daily Calorie Budget |
|---|---|---|
|  |  |  |
|  |  |  |
|  |  |  |
|  |  |  |
|  |  |  |
|  |  |  |
|  |  |  |
|  |  |  |
|  |  |  |
|  |  |  |
|  |  |  |

CHAPTER 7

# COOKING WITH CALORIES IN MIND

# CREATE YOUR RECIPE CARDS

*The secret to success here is to build your meal plans around foods you love and enjoy. Create meals to your taste without losing sight of your end goal – balancing nutrients and keeping your calories down. REMEMBER: You don't need to be a professional chef to do this.*

+ Personalise recipes and cook meals that work for you and fit around your life.

+ Use the following recipe card templates to document some of your favourite new recipes.

+ There is a perception that healthy eating is expensive, but that is another myth we need to burst. Use the recipe cost calculator on the reverse page of each recipe card to work out the cost per serving for your recipe.

## RECIPE FOR .................................................................................
*(name of the dish)*

Prep time: ..................................... Serves: ...................................
*(number of servings)*

Cooking time: ............ Calories per serve: ............ Cost per serving: ............

Ingredients:

..................................................... .....................................................

..................................................... .....................................................

..................................................... .....................................................

..................................................... .....................................................

..................................................... .....................................................

..................................................... .....................................................

Method:

.......................................................................................................

.......................................................................................................

.......................................................................................................

.......................................................................................................

.......................................................................................................

.......................................................................................................

.......................................................................................................

.......................................................................................................

.......................................................................................................

.......................................................................................................

# RECIPE COST CALCULATOR

**Recipe Name:** ........................................................................................................

| Ingredient Name | Quantity Purchased | Cost | Quantity used in recipe | Cost |
|---|---|---|---|---|
|  |  |  |  |  |
|  |  |  |  |  |
|  |  |  |  |  |
|  |  |  |  |  |
|  |  |  |  |  |
|  |  |  |  |  |
|  |  |  |  |  |
|  |  |  |  |  |
|  |  |  |  |  |
|  |  |  |  |  |
|  |  |  |  |  |

*Total cost per batch*

*Number of servings*

*Cost per serving*
*(total cost divided by number of servings)*

## RECIPE FOR ...........................................................................................
*(name of the dish)*

Prep time: ........................................... Serves: ..........................................
*(number of servings)*

Cooking time: ............ Calories per serve: ............ Cost per serving: ............

### Ingredients:

........................................................  ........................................................

........................................................  ........................................................

........................................................  ........................................................

........................................................  ........................................................

........................................................  ........................................................

........................................................  ........................................................

### Method:

....................................................................................................................

....................................................................................................................

....................................................................................................................

....................................................................................................................

....................................................................................................................

....................................................................................................................

....................................................................................................................

....................................................................................................................

....................................................................................................................

....................................................................................................................

....................................................................................................................

# RECIPE COST CALCULATOR

**Recipe Name:** .............................................................................................................

| Ingredient Name | Quantity Purchased | Cost | Quantity used in recipe | Cost |
|---|---|---|---|---|
| | | | | |
| | | | | |
| | | | | |
| | | | | |
| | | | | |
| | | | | |
| | | | | |
| | | | | |
| | | | | |
| | | | | |
| | | | | |

*Total cost per batch*

*Number of servings*

*Cost per serving*
*(total cost divided by number of servings)*

## RECIPE FOR ...............................................................................................................
*(name of the dish)*

Prep time: ................................................ Serves: ..............................................
*(number of servings)*

Cooking time: ............. Calories per serve: .............. Cost per serving: ..............

## Ingredients:

..................................................      ..................................................

..................................................      ..................................................

..................................................      ..................................................

..................................................      ..................................................

..................................................      ..................................................

..................................................      ..................................................

## Method:

..............................................................................................................................

..............................................................................................................................

..............................................................................................................................

..............................................................................................................................

..............................................................................................................................

..............................................................................................................................

..............................................................................................................................

..............................................................................................................................

..............................................................................................................................

..............................................................................................................................

# RECIPE COST CALCULATOR

**Recipe Name:** ...........................................................................................................

| Ingredient Name | Quantity Purchased | Cost | Quantity used in recipe | Cost |
|---|---|---|---|---|
|  |  |  |  |  |
|  |  |  |  |  |
|  |  |  |  |  |
|  |  |  |  |  |
|  |  |  |  |  |
|  |  |  |  |  |
|  |  |  |  |  |
|  |  |  |  |  |
|  |  |  |  |  |
|  |  |  |  |  |
|  |  |  |  |  |

*Total cost per batch*

*Number of servings*

*Cost per serving*
*(total cost divided by number of servings)*

**RECIPE FOR** ...........................................................................................................
*(name of the dish)*

Prep time: ................................................ Serves: ....................................................
*(number of servings)*

Cooking time: ............ Calories per serve: ............ Cost per serving: ............

Ingredients:

........................................................     ........................................................

........................................................     ........................................................

........................................................     ........................................................

........................................................     ........................................................

........................................................     ........................................................

........................................................     ........................................................

Method:

............................................................................................................................

............................................................................................................................

............................................................................................................................

............................................................................................................................

............................................................................................................................

............................................................................................................................

............................................................................................................................

............................................................................................................................

............................................................................................................................

............................................................................................................................

## RECIPE COST CALCULATOR

**Recipe Name:** ................................................................................................................

| Ingredient Name | Quantity Purchased | Cost | Quantity used in recipe | Cost |
|---|---|---|---|---|
|  |  |  |  |  |
|  |  |  |  |  |
|  |  |  |  |  |
|  |  |  |  |  |
|  |  |  |  |  |
|  |  |  |  |  |
|  |  |  |  |  |
|  |  |  |  |  |
|  |  |  |  |  |
|  |  |  |  |  |
|  |  |  |  |  |

*Total cost per batch*

*Number of servings*

*Cost per serving*
*(total cost divided by number of servings)*

**RECIPE FOR** ......................................................................................
*(name of the dish)*

Prep time: ................................... Serves: ...........................................
*(number of servings)*

Cooking time: ............. Calories per serve: ............. Cost per serving: .............

Ingredients:

..................................................          ..................................................

..................................................          ..................................................

..................................................          ..................................................

..................................................          ..................................................

..................................................          ..................................................

..................................................          ..................................................

Method:

........................................................................................................

........................................................................................................

........................................................................................................

........................................................................................................

........................................................................................................

........................................................................................................

........................................................................................................

........................................................................................................

........................................................................................................

........................................................................................................

........................................................................................................

# RECIPE COST CALCULATOR

**Recipe Name:** ................................................................................................................

| Ingredient Name | Quantity Purchased | Cost | Quantity used in recipe | Cost |
|---|---|---|---|---|
| | | | | |
| | | | | |
| | | | | |
| | | | | |
| | | | | |
| | | | | |
| | | | | |
| | | | | |
| | | | | |
| | | | | |
| | | | | |

*Total cost per batch*

*Number of servings*

*Cost per serving*
*(total cost divided by number of servings)*

# RECIPE FOR .........................................................................
*(name of the dish)*

Prep time: .................................... Serves: ...............................................
*(number of servings)*

Cooking time: ............. Calories per serve: ............. Cost per serving: .............

## Ingredients:

....................................................     ....................................................

....................................................     ....................................................

....................................................     ....................................................

....................................................     ....................................................

....................................................     ....................................................

....................................................     ....................................................

## Method:

..........................................................................................................................

..........................................................................................................................

..........................................................................................................................

..........................................................................................................................

..........................................................................................................................

..........................................................................................................................

..........................................................................................................................

..........................................................................................................................

..........................................................................................................................

..........................................................................................................................

# RECIPE COST CALCULATOR

**Recipe Name:** ........................................................................................

| Ingredient Name | Quantity Purchased | Cost | Quantity used in recipe | Cost |
|---|---|---|---|---|
|  |  |  |  |  |
|  |  |  |  |  |
|  |  |  |  |  |
|  |  |  |  |  |
|  |  |  |  |  |
|  |  |  |  |  |
|  |  |  |  |  |
|  |  |  |  |  |
|  |  |  |  |  |
|  |  |  |  |  |
|  |  |  |  |  |

*Total cost per batch*

*Number of servings*

*Cost per serving*
*(total cost divided by number of servings)*

# RECIPE FOR .........................................................................................
*(name of the dish)*

Prep time: .............................................. Serves: ..................................................
*(number of servings)*

Cooking time: ............ Calories per serve: ............ Cost per serving: ............

Ingredients:

........................................................    ........................................................

........................................................    ........................................................

........................................................    ........................................................

........................................................    ........................................................

........................................................    ........................................................

........................................................    ........................................................

Method:

.....................................................................................................................

.....................................................................................................................

.....................................................................................................................

.....................................................................................................................

.....................................................................................................................

.....................................................................................................................

.....................................................................................................................

.....................................................................................................................

.....................................................................................................................

.....................................................................................................................

# RECIPE COST CALCULATOR

**Recipe Name:** ..............................................................................................................

| Ingredient Name | Quantity Purchased | Cost | Quantity used in recipe | Cost |
|---|---|---|---|---|
|  |  |  |  |  |
|  |  |  |  |  |
|  |  |  |  |  |
|  |  |  |  |  |
|  |  |  |  |  |
|  |  |  |  |  |
|  |  |  |  |  |
|  |  |  |  |  |
|  |  |  |  |  |
|  |  |  |  |  |
|  |  |  |  |  |

*Total cost per batch*

*Number of servings*

*Cost per serving*
*(total cost divided by number of servings)*

## RECIPE FOR......................................................................................

*(name of the dish)*

Prep time: .............................................. Serves: ..........................................

*(number of servings)*

Cooking time: ............. Calories per serve: ............. Cost per serving: .............

## Ingredients:

........................................................... ...........................................................

........................................................... ...........................................................

........................................................... ...........................................................

........................................................... ...........................................................

........................................................... ...........................................................

........................................................... ...........................................................

## Method:

...................................................................................................................

...................................................................................................................

...................................................................................................................

...................................................................................................................

...................................................................................................................

...................................................................................................................

...................................................................................................................

...................................................................................................................

...................................................................................................................

...................................................................................................................

...................................................................................................................

## RECIPE COST CALCULATOR

**Recipe Name:** ...........................................................................................................

| Ingredient Name | Quantity Purchased | Cost | Quantity used in recipe | Cost |
|---|---|---|---|---|
|  |  |  |  |  |
|  |  |  |  |  |
|  |  |  |  |  |
|  |  |  |  |  |
|  |  |  |  |  |
|  |  |  |  |  |
|  |  |  |  |  |
|  |  |  |  |  |
|  |  |  |  |  |
|  |  |  |  |  |
|  |  |  |  |  |

*Total cost per batch*

*Number of servings*

*Cost per serving*
*(total cost divided by number of servings)*

**RECIPE FOR** .............................................................................................................
*(name of the dish)*

Prep time: .................................... Serves: ........................................
*(number of servings)*

Cooking time: ............ Calories per serve: ............ Cost per serving: ............

Ingredients:

......................................................    ......................................................
......................................................    ......................................................
......................................................    ......................................................
......................................................    ......................................................
......................................................    ......................................................
......................................................    ......................................................

Method:

.................................................................................................................
.................................................................................................................
.................................................................................................................
.................................................................................................................
.................................................................................................................
.................................................................................................................
.................................................................................................................
.................................................................................................................
.................................................................................................................
.................................................................................................................

# RECIPE COST CALCULATOR

**Recipe Name:** ...........................................................................................................

| Ingredient Name | Quantity Purchased | Cost | Quantity used in recipe | Cost |
|---|---|---|---|---|
|  |  |  |  |  |
|  |  |  |  |  |
|  |  |  |  |  |
|  |  |  |  |  |
|  |  |  |  |  |
|  |  |  |  |  |
|  |  |  |  |  |
|  |  |  |  |  |
|  |  |  |  |  |
|  |  |  |  |  |
|  |  |  |  |  |

*Total cost per batch*

*Number of servings*

*Cost per serving*
*(total cost divided by number of servings)*

# RECIPE FOR
*(name of the dish)*

Prep time: ............................................. Serves: ...........................................
*(number of servings)*

Cooking time: ............ Calories per serve: ............ Cost per serving: ............

## Ingredients:

...........................................................  ...........................................................
...........................................................  ...........................................................
...........................................................  ...........................................................
...........................................................  ...........................................................
...........................................................  ...........................................................
...........................................................  ...........................................................

## Method:

...................................................................................................................
...................................................................................................................
...................................................................................................................
...................................................................................................................
...................................................................................................................
...................................................................................................................
...................................................................................................................
...................................................................................................................
...................................................................................................................
...................................................................................................................
...................................................................................................................

# RECIPE COST CALCULATOR

**Recipe Name:** ..........................................................................................................

| Ingredient Name | Quantity Purchased | Cost | Quantity used in recipe | Cost |
|---|---|---|---|---|
|  |  |  |  |  |
|  |  |  |  |  |
|  |  |  |  |  |
|  |  |  |  |  |
|  |  |  |  |  |
|  |  |  |  |  |
|  |  |  |  |  |
|  |  |  |  |  |
|  |  |  |  |  |
|  |  |  |  |  |
|  |  |  |  |  |

*Total cost per batch*

*Number of servings*

*Cost per serving*
*(total cost divided by number of servings)*

# MEAL PLANNING

+ Use the meal plan template to build a go-to 1-week meal plan based on:

    + Low calorie meals that were enjoyable and filling.
    + Meals that consistently feature on days you keep total calories lower than your budget.
    + Exercise routines/activity that helped you to burn more calories.

+ This meal plan will come in handy when you occasionally get off track and need to regain control of your weight.

# MY FAIL-SAFE MEAL PLAN

| Day /Date | Breakfast ............ kcal | Lunch ............ kcal | Dinner ............ kcal | Snacks ............ kcal |
|---|---|---|---|---|
| | Calorie budget ............ kcal | | Exercise/ Steps ............ kcal | Calorie Balance/deficit ............ kcal |
| Day /Date | Breakfast ............ kcal | Lunch ............ kcal | Dinner ............ kcal | Snacks ............ kcal |
| | Calorie budget ............ kcal | | Exercise/ Steps ............ kcal | Calorie Balance/deficit ............ kcal |
| Day /Date | Breakfast ............ kcal | Lunch ............ kcal | Dinner ............ kcal | Snacks ............ kcal |
| | Calorie budget ............ kcal | | Exercise/ Steps ............ kcal | Calorie Balance/deficit ............ kcal |
| Day /Date | Breakfast ............ kcal | Lunch ............ kcal | Dinner ............ kcal | Snacks ............ kcal |
| | Calorie budget ............ kcal | | Exercise/ Steps ............ kcal | Calorie Balance/deficit ............ kcal |
| Day /Date | Breakfast ............ kcal | Lunch ............ kcal | Dinner ............ kcal | Snacks ............ kcal |
| | Calorie budget ............ kcal | | Exercise/ Steps ............ kcal | Calorie Balance/deficit ............ kcal |
| Day /Date | Breakfast ............ kcal | Lunch ............ kcal | Dinner ............ kcal | Snacks ............ kcal |
| | Calorie budget ............ kcal | | Exercise/ Steps ............ kcal | Calorie Balance/deficit ............ kcal |
| Day /Date | Breakfast ............ kcal | Lunch ............ kcal | Dinner ............ kcal | Snacks ............ kcal |
| | Calorie budget ............ kcal | | Exercise/ Steps ............ kcal | Calorie Balance/deficit ............ kcal |

# CHAPTER 8

# MEASURE IT TO MANAGE IT

*As is said in management, you cannot manage what you do not measure. While eating well may seem the most crucial, the only way to know that you are doing so is by measuring what you consume. By measuring, you can easily assess the impact on your body weight and the other parameters.*

*If you are using an app, it probably does the performance tracking and generates these charts automatically. Otherwise, you can do this manually using the next few trackers.*

*Quality data produces quality insights and helps you to make quality decisions about your plan going forward.*

## WEIGHT TRACKER (KILOGRAMS)

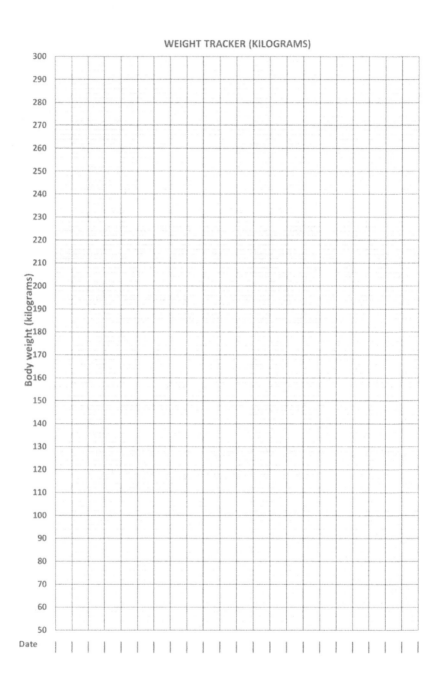

## WEIGHT TRACKER (POUNDS)

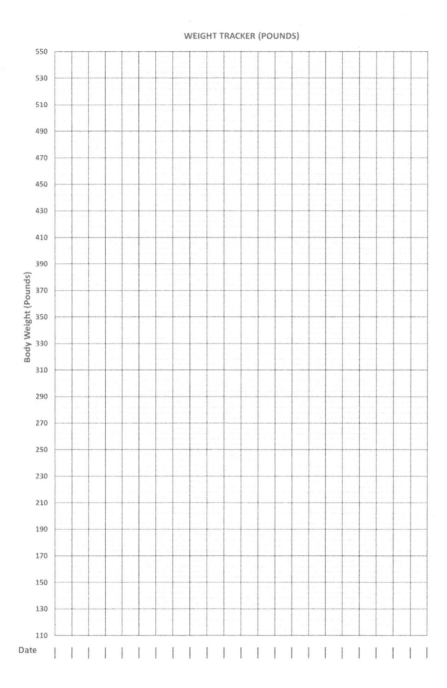

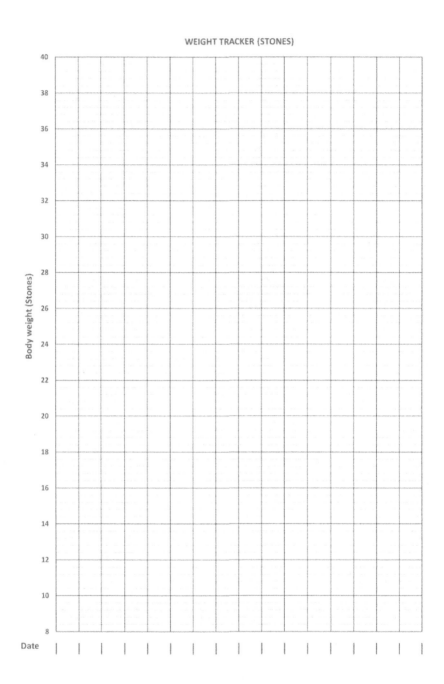

## Bicep|Chest|Hip|Neck|Thigh|Waist Measurement
(colour code if needed. e.g. red for hips, blue for waist.)

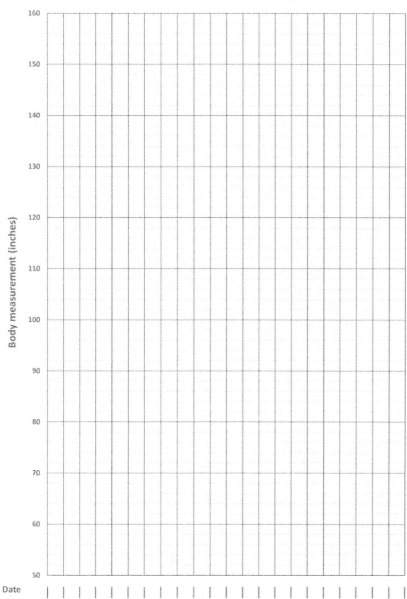

Body measurement (inches)

Date

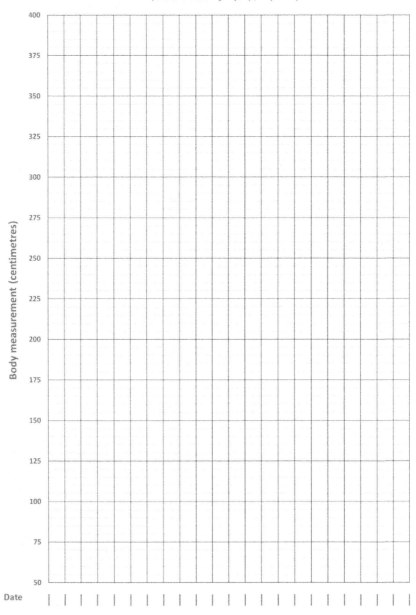

# A NEW NORMAL - YOUR NEXT STEP

Well done for coming this far. You have not only developed your own comprehensive, personalised weight loss plan without a personal trainer, but you have also started to implement your plan, and hopefully started to see the results.

I'd love to see you continue your weight loss journey, achieve your goal, and keep the weight off for life. So, stick to your plan and keep tracking and measuring.

You can continue to do this with your weight loss app. However, if you choose to track your progress manually, I recommend that you use the 'Weight Loss Code Breaker - 90 Days Calorie Control Journal'.

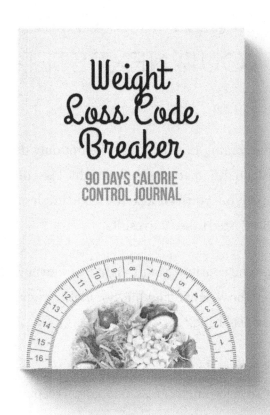

Get your journal now on

*Amazon*

OR

*www.weightlosscode.co.uk*

## REVIEWS MAKE A WRITER'S WORLD GO ROUND

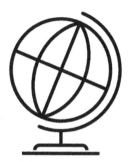

**Thank you for reading my book!**

I really appreciate all your feedback, and I love hearing what you have to say.

I need your input to make the next version of this book and my future books better.

Kindly leave me a helpful review on Amazon or any of the other marketplaces where you purchased my book and let me know what you thought of it.

Thank you so much!


-Yemi Fadipe

# NOTES

Made in the USA
Monee, IL
23 April 2021